Natural Treatments for Depression

2nd Edition

C.M. Hawken

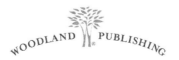

WOODLAND PUBLISHING

For permissions, ordering information, or bulk quantity discounts, contact:
Woodland Publishing, Salt Lake City, Utah
Visit our Web site: www.woodlandpublishing.com
Toll-free number: (800) 777-BOOK

The information in this book is for educational purposes only and is not recommended as a means of diagnosing or treating an illness. All matters concerning physical and mental health should be supervised by a health practitioner knowledgeable in treating that particular condition. Neither the publisher nor the author directly or indirectly dispenses medical advice, nor do they prescribe any remedies or assume any responsibility for those who choose to treat themselves.

Cataloging-in-Publication data is available from the Library of Congress.

ISBN-13: 978-1-58054-190-9

Printed in the United States of America

Contents

Depression: An Overview

Depression affects millions of people worldwide. It is one of the most common psychiatric complaints, and physicians have described it since the time of Hippocrates, who called it "melancholia." In 2010, the National Institute of Mental Health reported that depression and mood disorders affect nearly 10 percent of American adults through all racial, economic and social groups. These disorders take many forms, but they are usually

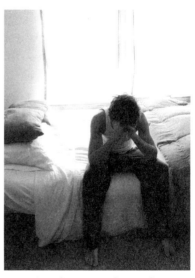

Depression takes on many forms and affects millions of adults.

marked by sadness, inactivity and self-depreciation. Hopelessness and pessimism are common symptoms of depression, as are lowered self-esteem, reduced energy and vitality and loss of overall enjoyment.

The effects of depression vary widely. Depression may be short term, it may recur repeatedly at short intervals or it may be somewhat permanent. It can be mild or severe, acute or chronic. Reported rates of incidence are two to three times higher among women than men. Men are more likely to suffer from depression as they grow older, while women are most likely to suffer from depression between the ages of 35 and 45.

Depression has many causes. These can include childhood traumas, physical disorders, overly stressful situations at work or at home, biochemical processes, diet, illness, drug use, stressful life events and more. For instance, defective regulation of the release of one or more organic compounds in the brain called *amines*—particularly norepinephrine, serotonin and dopamine—leads to reduced quantities of these chemicals, bringing about depression. Some health experts suggest that underlying conditions like diabetes or cancer can cause depression. Others suggest that acute stress can trigger or worsen depression. And others point to simple causes—such as lack of exercise—that, when remedied, can relieve symptoms of depression.

Types of Depression

Life often presents situations and events that can make us feel down, perhaps even desperate and hopeless. But such feelings are normal under certain circumstances. Only when these episodes become extreme, last for long periods or overcome a person's life do doctors typically diagnose depression.

There are several different types of depression. For the purposes of this booklet we refer to mild to moderate levels of depression, known as dysthymia, the most common type of depression. Other forms of depression include major depression (bi-polar disorder, manic depression), post-stroke depression, seasonal affective disorder (SAD) and post-partum depression.

Clinical Depression (Dysthymia)

According to the American Psychiatric Association (APA), the symptoms of clinical depression, or dysthymia, include the following:

1. Poor appetite with weight loss, or increased appetite with weight gain
2. Physical hyperactivity or inactivity
3. Loss of interest or pleasure in usual activities
4. Decreased sex drive
5. Insomnia or hypersomnia (excessive sleeping)
6. Feelings of worthlessness, self-reproach or inappropriate guilt
7. Diminished ability to think or concentrate
8. Recurrent thoughts of death or suicide

According to the APA's *Diagnostic and Statistical Manual of Mental Disorders* (DSM-IV), a person must experience five of these eight symptoms to qualify as depressed. However, many health experts state that the severity and length of any of these symptoms can indicate depression.

Seasonal Affective Disorder (SAD)

Long winters can take a toll on the hardiest soul: short days and long nights, being stuck indoors, shoveling snow, scraping cars and occasionally slipping on the ice can be wearying. But what happens when the winter blues become something more serious?

Though the etiology is unclear, physicians increasingly admit there is a close link between decreased winter sunlight and increased complaints of general depressive symptoms. But while this seasonal variation affects some people profoundly, others it does not affect at all.

Seasonal winter depression is known as seasonal affective disorder (SAD). So far, the exact cause of SAD is unknown. Some researchers attribute it to decreased melatonin levels, which play a crucial role in circadian rhythms; some blame decreased levels of serotonin caused by a lack of sunlight; some think the key hormone is catecholamine, which is central to the body's "fight or flight" reaction, and that sunlight is necessary to keep it at a normal level; others argue that SAD results from a combination of some or all of the above and perhaps some other factors not yet discovered.

The most common treatment for SAD is light therapy. If going outside to soak up the sun is impossible or insufficient, special lamps that mimic natural sunlight have proven highly effective in combating SAD. The patient should sit in front (or slightly to the side) of the light for up to one hour each morning. Light therapy can be combined with many daily activities, such as eating, working on the computer and reading.

Postpartum Depression (PPD)

Postpartum depression is a common complication of childbirth. More severe than the "baby blues," postpartum depression interferes with a mother's life and her ability to care for her new baby. A woman's hormones fluctuate wildly immediately after childbirth, and her emotions can go along for the ride. A small emotional letdown is normal, and the lack of sleep can take a toll on the hardiest of women. But if the depression begins to affect a woman's daily life and her baby, it is important to talk to someone: her midwife or doctor, her partner, her friends or other women who have experienced childbirth.

Estrogen therapy is used to relieve menopausal symptoms, but it can also help stabilize postpartum mood swings. Because estrogen therapy targets hormonal imbalances, it specifically targets the cause of the postpartum depression.

Other therapies can help relieve postpartum depression. Light therapy, which is usually used to relieve seasonal affective disorder, can complement other treatments for postpartum depression. Preliminary studies have shown promising results for omega-3 fatty acids, and some researchers recommend carbohydrate-rich diets in conjunction with the methods described above. Counseling and support groups may also help women overcome postpartum depression. For more information on PPD, see the appendix on page 30.

Treating Depression

Natural treatments for depression have become more common lately, giving people with depression more tools to fight their condition. The emergence of natural treatments is especially important because diagnoses of depression are increasing each year. As diagnoses of depression increase, so too has the prevalence of drugs designed to treat depression. This booklet discusses the various treatments for depression in order to illuminate the value of natural and alternative treatments.

Standard Treatments for Depression

Health practitioners have many tools for treating depression and other nervous disorders. The two most common are psychotherapy and drug therapy.

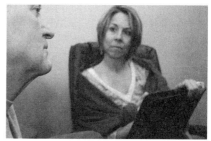

Cognitive behavioral therapy is a conventional treatment for depression.

Psychotherapy (also known as cognitive behavioral therapy) aims to resolve underlying psychic conflicts that may cause depression and to give emotional support to the patient. Psychotherapy usually involves regular visits to a psychiatrist or a psychologist and may also include participation in support groups. Research indicates that psychotherapy can help people deal effectively with depression, but results can be sporadic and short-lived.

Antidepressant drugs, on the other hand, directly affect chemicals in the brain called monoamines, which likely play an important part in mood. The most common antidepressants fall into two categories: selective serotonin reuptake inhibitors (SSRIs) and monoamine oxidase inhibitors (MAOIs).

SSRIs are perhaps the most well known antidepressants and include brands such as Prozac, Celexa, Paxil, Zoloft and Lexapro. Scientists suggest they work by increasing the life of monoamine transmitters, allowing these neurotransmitters to accumulate in the brain and remain in contact with nerve cell receptors longer, thus helping to elevate the patient's mood.

MAOIs inhibit the activity of an enzyme called oxidase, which breaks down the monoamine neurotransmitters and results in reduced levels of serotonin, norepinephrine and epinephrine. While SSRIs increase the life of monoamines, MAOIs increase the availability of monoamines.

Randomized controlled trials show that many drugs not normally considered antidepressants—including benzodiazepenes, opiates, busiprone, stimulants, reserpine, and antipsychotics—can have effects similar to those of antidepressants, suggesting that a placebo effect may be responsible for some of the benefits of antidepressants. Also, many patients who take antidepressants experience undesirable side effects, including nausea, bloating, indigestion, abdominal cramping, diarrhea and other gastrointestinal discomforts. Dizziness is another common complaint, as are mouth dryness, heart problems, sexual side effects and more.

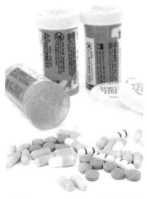

Antidepressant drugs alter brain chemistry and may have negative side effects.

Standard Antidepressant Drugs

MAOIs

Monoamine oxidase inhibitors (MAOIs) are the original antidepressants. They relieve symptoms of depression by inhibiting the enzyme monoamine oxidase, which is responsible for breaking down serotonin and other chemical compounds in the brain. MAOIs allow for increased production of these neurotransmitters, ultimately resulting in elevated mood levels. Because their primary effect is to stimulate rather than sedate,

MAOIs can easily cause insomnia, inability to focus and problems with coordination, as well as more typical side effects like dry mouth, gastrointestinal problems and dizziness. These side effects, however, are mild. Serious conditions, such as excessively high blood pressure and brain hemorrhage, can occur if a person takes MAOIs with certain over-the-counter cold and cough remedies or with certain foods, such as cheese, dried meats, wine and concentrated yeast products.

SSRIs

Selective serotonin reuptake inhibitors (SSRIs) increase the amount of serotonin in the brain by inhibiting the serotonin reuptake process, thus keeping serotonin in contact with the nerves longer. Fluoxetine (Prozac), the first SSRI, was introduced to the medical world in 1987 and immediately dominated the American antidepressant market. (Other SSRIs have since appeared under different brand names.) Sales of Prozac peaked at $2.8 billion in 2001, when the generic equivalent was introduced. In 2008, more than 2.2 million fluoxetine prescriptions were filled.

Though generally considered safe, fluoxetine may cause side effects such as insomnia, anxiety and restlessness; indicating, in other words, that fluoxetine is too much of an "upper." Fluoxetine has also been linked to different forms of destructive, if not bizarre, behavior. Researchers have documented cases linking the drug to suicide. Other side effects of fluoxetine may include headaches, nausea, weight fluctuation and dry mouth.

Tricyclic Antidepressants

Before the emergence of Prozac, physicians prescribed tricyclic antidepressants for most cases of major depression and dysthymia. Tricyclic antidepressants decrease the occurrence of depressive symptoms by encouraging the activity of neurotransmitters in the brain and the nervous system. Despite being widely prescribed, these drugs can cause a number of adverse side effects, including dry mouth, constipation and other gastrointestinal problems, dizziness, increased appetite (and subsequent weight gain) and blurred vision.

Alternative Treatments for Depression

Because of the complexity of depression doctors and patients often have difficulty determining the ideal course of treatment. Many people are reluctant to use antidepressant drugs because of their side effects, and instead prefer natural or alternative treatments such as herbs and supplements. The following are some of the most common and effective supplements for treating various forms of depression.

St. John's Wort *(Hypericum perforatum)*

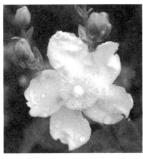

St. John's wort is a traditional herbal remedy for depression.

One of the most effective herbal remedies for depression is St. John's wort, an herb also known as hypericum. St. John's wort has simple, whorled, gland-dotted leaves that are usually smooth margined. Its flowers are yellow and have five petals and many stamens, often in bundles.

St. John's wort grows in many areas around the world, from Australia to Europe to the United States, and it grows especially well in Northern California and Oregon. The plant supposedly received the name *St. John's wort* because it flowers around the time of St. John's Eve, June 23. The word *wort* comes from the Old English term *wyrt*, which means plant, herb or vegetable.

Folk medicine practitioners have historically used hypericum to treat many problems, including mood disorders and depression. The first recorded use of St. John's wort occurred during the Crusades, when people used it to treat battle wounds and enhance mental alertness. St. John's wort was also used to treat insanity and mental instability, and it was even used to treat the supposed "possessions" and hallucinations of witches. Contemporary research supports these uses and suggests that St. John's wort supports the healing of topical wounds and treats disorders of "mood and temperament."

While the popularity of hypericum is limited to the peripheral areas of health care in the United States, the plant's use in Europe and other parts of the world justify calling hypericum a mainstream treatment. In Germany, St. John's wort extracts are licensed for the treatment of anxiety, depression and sleep disorders and are commonly given to children and teenagers. Reports estimate that hypericum prescriptions constitute nearly half of the German antidepressant market.

Randomized clinical trials have compared the effects of pharmaceutical preparations of hypericum with those of placebos and common antidepressants. Nearly all of the studies favored hypericum treatments for mild to moderate depression and related disorders. These studies also showed that hypericum causes significantly fewer side effects than synthetic drugs; in some studies, researchers attributed fewer side effects to hypericum than they did to a placebo.

One may wonder why it is only relatively recently that Americans are being exposed to St. John's wort. There are several probable reasons for this (including our society's condescending attitude toward natural therapies and the medical profession's unwillingness to trust the research on hypericum), but they are a topic for another book. The important thing to remember is that research supports the use of hypericum as an effective and affordable treatment for depression with fewer side effects than synthetic drugs.

How St. John's Wort Works

Scientists suggest that hypericin, first isolated from St. John's wort in 1942, may be the major compound with antidepressant properties. However, evidence for this still remains inconclusive as the exact mechanism of action eludes researchers. Long-term use of a hypericum extract containing hypericin suggests that it did modify levels of neurotransmitters in the parts of the brain involved with the expression of depression. The study also concluded that it was less effective in the short term.

The second active compound, hyperforin, is a newer compound being studied for its antidepressant activities. A study suggests that hyperforin is the major fat-soluble component that acts as un uptake inhibitor of serotonin, dopamine, noradrenaline, GABA and L-Glutamate, meaning that it keeps these major "feel good" neurotransmitters in the synapses longer and that this may be its possible antidepressant action. The experiment was also done with pure hyperforin with equally positive results. This research is a starting point for new drug projects.

Research Concerning St. John's Wort and Depression

Many studies have compared hypericum extract to placebos and standard antidepressants, including their effects on mild and moderate forms of major depression and the scope and severity of their side effects. One such study, which was instrumental in bringing hypericum to the public's attention, was published in the *British Medical Journal* in 1996.

The researchers behind this study showed hypericum extracts to be "significantly superior" to a placebo and similarly effective to standard antidepressants. Percentage-wise, twice as many patients taking standard antidepressant drugs dropped out of the study due to side effects compared to those taking hypericum extracts.

The researchers evaluated the patients using the Hamilton Depression Scale, a standard measure of depression. Patients taking hypericum treatments scored slightly better than those taking antidepressants and significantly better than those taking the placebo. (More recent studies suggest that St. John's wort is comparable to Prozac in effectiveness while producing fewer side effects.)

This study points strongly to the possibility of wide-scale use of St. John's wort to treat depression, especially since many people with depression are very concerned about side effects of pharmaceutical treatments and one of St. John's wort's most valuable assets is its relative lack thereof. The authors note that more research is necessary, especially to determine the severity and nature of depression that can be treated, the length of treatment, the proper dosage, the required strength of hypericum extracts and the potential for long-term side effects. Nevertheless, the results of this study and many others are promising for the millions of people who suffer from depression.

As previously mentioned, many studies have compared the effects of hypericum on depression with those of placebos and other standard drug therapies. Here are some points of interest from these studies:

In several of the studies, the number of subjects who dropped out (due to side effects) was nearly identical in the placebo group and in the hypericum group. In some studies, there were more dropouts in the placebo group than in the hypericum group. In most studies, significantly more patients dropped out among those taking antidepressant drugs than among the patients taking hypericum extracts. This supports the argument that hypericum extracts cause few (if any) undesirable side effects, which is of principal concern to most people with depression.

Many of the studies note that patients taking hypericum are much more likely to be "very much improved" or "no longer ill;" that is, after treatment with hypericum they no longer experience enough symptoms to qualify as depressed under various depression rating systems. This indicates that hypericum may be capable of completely relieving depression.

Because many early studies on hypericum focused on subjects with only mild to moderate depression, hypericum was not recommended for patients suffering from severe major depression. However, more recent studies show hypericum to outperform imipramine in patients with severe depression (imipramine is a standard antidepressant used to treat severe depression). Another study demonstrated that the effects of hypericum and fluoxetine (Prozac) on moderate to severe depression were almost the same and that the patients tolerated hypericum much better.

Recent studies suggest that St. John's wort can treat obsessive-compulsive disorder, generalized anxiety disorder and alcohol dependence.

Several studies (and commentary by researchers) suggest that hypericum has a cumulative effect, becoming more and more effective the longer it is used.

Researchers in all of these studies recommend that hypericum be considered a viable option for treating mild to moderate depression, citing hypericum's broad range of therapeutic activity, its relative lack of side effects and its excellent treatment record. (Interestingly, many of these researchers are trained in standard medicine, not natural or herbal medicine, and are not necessarily sympathetic to alternative treatments.)

Please note: Patients who take blood thinners or other antidepressants should not take St. John's wort, as interactions can cause strokes. St. John's wort can also reduce the effectiveness of oral contraceptives. Please consult a healthcare practitioner before starting any form of treatment.

Other Natural Treatments for Depression

Besides St. John's wort, natural treatments for depression include other herbal supplements, diet, exercise and more. Some treatments, including the herb valerian, have been tested in combination with St. John's wort. The following is a discussion of several promising complementary therapies. To determine if any are right for you, consult with a doctor of osteopathy, a chiropractor or a naturopathic physician.

Valerian Root (*Valeriana officinalis*)

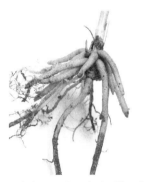

Valerian has long been used to treat nervous disorders such as depression, insomnia and anxiety. Valerian sedative effects have been well documented; two of this country's major medical registers, the *U.S. Pharmacopeia* and the *U.S. Formulary*, list valerian as a tranquilizing agent. In addition, research shows valerian may combat hormonal instabilities and alleviate symptoms of premenstrual syndrome and postmenopause.

Valerian root is an herb with well-documented sedative effects.

Valerian relieves insomnia and improves sleep by relaxing smooth muscle and inhibiting processes of the nervous system, thereby promoting a calm feeling and deeper, more restful sleep. Valerian does not cause sluggishness or grogginess, which are common side effects of tranquilizer-like drugs used to promote sleep.

5-HTP (5-hydroxytryptophan)

5-HTP is the raw material the body uses to make serotonin, a key neurotransmitter that maintains mood levels in the brain. The body produces 5-HTP from tryptophan, a naturally occurring amino acid. Although the role of 5-HTP in serotonin production has been recognized for years, only recently have American doctors and consumers begun focusing on 5-HTP as a treatment for depression and other mood disorders.

Researchers began investigating 5-HTP and its possible therapeutic capabilities in the 1960s. Early on, they discovered that 5-HTP was quickly converted into serotonin. But the lack of research led these researchers to wonder about 5-HTP's safety, its application for humans and its possible side effects.

Consequently, new studies investigated how 5-HTP worked and whether it was safe. One of the first of these studies was conducted in Japan and involved patients suffering from either unipolar depression or bipolar depression (the most severe form of depression). Within approximately two weeks, more than 50 percent of the patients experienced some improvement in their symptoms; when the four-week trial was concluded, almost 75 percent of the patients indicated they had experienced complete relief of their symptoms or at least significant improvement.

Since the initial studies carried in Japan, more research has been done but recent research indicates that more studies are still needed. Though preliminary studies suggest that 5-HTP is more effective than a placebo, many studies aren't of high enough quality to be reliable. At present, we cannot say definitively that 5-HTP is an effective treatment for depression.

Hops

Though very few studies have been performed on hops, the herb has historically been used as a mood stabilizer and natural sedative. In the 18th century, European field workers harvesting hops could rarely work a full day because they became so fatigued while working with the plant. Hops is a nervine herb, meaning it has a calming effect on nerves. Like other nervine herbs, hops is considered effective in promoting muscle relaxation and restful sleep, relieving other symptoms of insomnia and stabilizing moods. One possible explanation for the nervine properties of hops may be the plant's high B-vitamin content. B vitamins play a crucial role in maintaining various body systems; a deficiency in any of the B vitamins can cause a plethora of ailments directly related to the nervous system, including sleep disorders, depression and anxiety. However, researchers agree that long-term controlled studies are needed to assess the role of hops in treating depression.

Amino Acids

Amino acids are essential to overall health, and their role in mood disorders is becoming better known. Certain amino acids, including L-tryptophan (see discussion on 5-HTP), L-tyrosine and L-phenylalanine, help the body produce neurotransmitters called amines. If the body is deficient in these three amino acids, the consequence is a drop in neurotransmitter function and ultimately a drop in mood. These amino acids are useful for treating carbohydrate cravings in people with SAD and for raising levels of serotonin, dopamine and norepinephrine, possibly the three most crucial compounds for controlling mood levels.

Vitamins/Minerals

Research increasingly points to certain vitamin and mineral deficiencies as a cause of depression and other nervous disorders. Of particular concern are the B vitamins. Vitamin B_6 deficiencies have been linked to people with depression, including new mothers with abnormally low B_6 levels. Exactly why B_6 deficiencies cause or exaggerate depression is not known, but the statistics point to its being a factor—nearly 20 percent of all people with depression are also deficient in vitamin B_6. (People who take oral contraceptives or synthetic drugs or who ingest high levels of caffeine are also known to have depleted B_6 levels.) B vitamins such as B_3, B_{12} and B_1 are necessary for other physiological processes, including the production of essential amino acids, a central factor in controlling psychiatric states.

Some studies that found low levels of vitamin B_{12} in depression sufferers found that these same subjects have low levels of folate (folic acid). Scientists have also linked low blood levels of folic acid and vitamin B_{12} to depression and to poor responses to antidepressant treatments. In some studies, researchers enhanced depression treatments by pairing St. John's wort or fluoxetine with a folic acid supplement. Interestingly, two places with traditional diets high in folate (Hong Kong and Taiwan) have lower rates of depression.

Vitamin C plays a principal role in mood and nervous system management. Taking vitamin C with bioflavonoids supports synthesis of norepinephrine and serotonin, two major neurotransmitters. Bioflavonoids, which are found naturally in the rinds of citrus fruits, green peppers, tomatoes, broccoli, cherries and other common foods, help the body assimilate vitamin C, thereby enhancing vitamin C's mood-elevating capabilities.

Magnesium is a mineral linked to vitamin B_6 in serotonin production, and studies have linked low magnesium levels to depression. Magnesium-rich foods include legumes, nuts, whole grains and green vegetables.

Ginkgo Biloba

Ginkgo biloba is a popular herb used to enhance mental clarity and circulation in the brain and extremities. Ginkgo has been used in China for various purposes for thousands of years; its main purpose in traditional Chinese medicine is enhancing brain function and improving respiratory health.

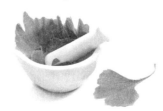

A large body of scientific research indicates that ginkgo improves circulation to the brain (and to the periph-

Ginkgo biloba may be a safe, natural alternative to pharmaceutical antidepressants.

eral areas of the body), thereby enhancing mental alertness and mood and giving a sense of more energy. Thus, ginkgo is widely used in Europe and other countries to treat cognitive impairment, and it is becoming increasingly popular in the United States.

Ginkgo is also being researched as a treatment for mild to moderate depression. Preliminary trials link ginkgo use to strong improvement in symptoms of depression, with virtually no side effects, suggesting that ginkgo may be a safe, natural alternative to antidepressant drugs.

Whom does ginkgo most help? The answer still isn't clear, but research indicates that ginkgo may inhibit the age-related loss of serotonin receptors; this suggests that older persons suffering from depression (which may be caused by the natural loss of serotonin receptors in the brain) may especially benefit from taking ginkgo.

Omega-3 Fatty Acids

Omega-3 fatty acids are essential for normal brain function. Recent studies have linked their intake (in conjunction with an antidepressant herb such as St. John's wort) to improvements in mood disorders such as bipolar disorder and major depression.

Although the body needs omega-3 fatty acids, it cannot produce them and must obtain them through diet. Omega-3 polyunsaturated fatty acids are found in high concentrations in fish such as salmon, sardines and anchovies. However, fish often contains mercury and other harmful chemicals, so many people prefer to get omega-3s from fish oil capsules, which are free of heavy metals. (Take fish oil capsules with a meal if you are concerned about a fishy aftertaste.)

Omega-3 fatty acids can interact with blood-thinning drugs such as warfarin and aspirin, so check with a doctor before taking omega-3 supplements.

SAM-e

S-adenosyl-L-methionine (SAM-e) is found naturally in all living cells and is believed to increase levels of serotonin and dopamine. Though research is still in the early stages, a small number of preliminary studies have been positive and controlled trials have found SAM-e to be more effective than placebos and as effective as tricyclic antidepressants for treating mood disorders. At this stage, researchers have performed more studies on SAM-e injections than on oral administrations of SAM-e.

Light Therapy and Seasonal Affective Disorder

Seasonal affective disorder (SAD) generally affects victims during the winter. As previously mentioned, the specific causes of SAD are unknown, but researchers believe that the key culprit is reduced sunlight.

Sunlight affects circadian rhythms and encourages the production of serotonin. Sunlight also provides the body with vitamin D, which the body needs to assimilate calcium. Studies correlate impaired absorption of vitamin D and calcium with the onset of depression, most notably SAD.

Because of the link between reduced sunlight and SAD, phototherapy, or light therapy, is a natural solution. Light therapy simply involves a patient sitting next to a specialized light box, which mimics natural sunlight. Studies show that light therapy usually relieves most people of the symptoms of depression.

Phototherapy has also been used to help people who work night shifts and to treat travelers suffering from jet lag.

In one study, researchers showed that phototherapy is especially effective when combined with hypericum therapy. The study showed that the hypericum extract helped SAD patients overcome a majority of their depressive symptoms. The researchers noted that hypericum may become a more popular treatment for SAD than phototherapy, because many patients consider phototherapy too time consuming.

Exercise

Exercise is extremely helpful for overcoming depression. Several studies indicate that exercise alone can dramatically improve one's mood levels and ability to handle stress. One recent study found that depressed subjects who participated in physical activities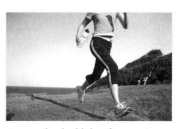

Among other health benefits, exercise can dramatically improve one's mood levels and ability to handle stress.

(such as sports and exercise) experienced a significant decrease in feelings of depression and malaise and fewer related ailments like insomnia.

Sleep Disturbances: Cause or Result of Depression?

It's a classic chicken-or-egg scenario: does insomnia cause depression, or does depression cause insomnia? Sales of prescription sleep medications have exploded in recent years along with the many new pills for depression. The pharmaceutical industry is aggressively marketing to the public with ads on television, on the Internet and more.

Anyone who has experienced chronic (or even occasional) insomnia knows its negative effects—headaches, irritability, inability to concentrate and daytime sleepiness (which may impair driving ability as much as alcohol) are just a few of its consequences. Some studies link insomnia to a two- to three-fold increase in paranoid thinking; paranoia and insomnia are in turn strongly associated with anxiety, worry, depression and irritability. Other studies indicate that insomnia may increase the risk of developing depression, increase the duration of depression and increase the chances of relapse following treatment of depression.

The Misdiagnosis of Depression

Too often, physicians will diagnose a person with depression-like symptoms as having depression, when in fact a physical disorder is causing or encouraging depression. This is a disturbing trend that raises several questions; for example, why are people being misdiagnosed and what about the undiscovered physical conditions?

Recent studies show that initial treatments for depression and mood disorders (both drug therapy and psychotherapy) have decreasing success rates. If we accept the idea that depression can be a symptom of another physical ailment, then treating the underlying physical disorder, not prescribing antidepressants, may be the best way of relieving depressive symptoms.

Is misdiagnosis really a problem? Several studies strongly suggest that physical disorders mimic psychiatric disorders or play an important role in their development—and it isn't a new trend. A 1979 study of 2,090 depressed subjects showed that 43 percent suffered from one or more physical illnesses, 46 percent of which were not diagnosed at the time of the original diagnosis of depression. A significant number of these patients were suffering from a major physical disorder that directly caused their symptoms of depression. A 1982 study provided strikingly similar results.

Although it has been more than 30 years since the first study was published, conditions have not improved. Recent papers call for a standardized physical exam for psychiatric patients, which does not currently exist. Currently, the quality of care patients receive depends entirely on their practitioner and the limits of his or her knowledge and experience. Without a standard in place, patients are subject to the luck of the draw. And, as author M.S. Gold points out in *The Hatherleigh Guide to Managing Depression,* health professionals, perform relatively poorly in diagnosing physical ailments when the ailment is accompanied by psychiatric symptoms.

The Relationship between Depression and Physical Disorders

Many conditions—including physical disorders, medications and drug or alcohol use—produce symptoms similar to those of depression. In fact, psychiatric symptoms are commonly the first signs of some reversible physical illness.

The presence of psychiatric symptoms, coupled with the way a health practitioner approaches the diagnosis, may be the primary causes of misdiagnosis. A doctor may lack knowledge, education or training; be unable to deal with physical illness; or be unwilling to incorporate new information into his or her practice. We should not hasten to malign physicians, however, as there are multiple reasons, most not the fault of the practitioner, that lead to misdiagnosis.

The problem of misdiagnosis was first brought to light in the previously mentioned 1979 study. The researchers found that less than 35 percent of the psychiatrists they polled performed any sort of physical exam (which could include simple questions as to other symptoms not related to depression or use of other medications, alcohol or drugs) on their subjects. The study found that even more of these doctors felt somewhat unable to perform a thorough physical.

Gold states that most mental health practitioners consult with the subject's general practitioner, specialist, gynecologist, etc. in place of performing a physical themselves. Admittedly, this is better than nothing; nevertheless, both medical and psychiatric professionals were generally poor at correctly diagnosing physical ailments when accompanied by depression and other psychiatric symptoms. And in the absence of a standardized test, this is not likely to have improved, even 30 years later, and doctors are still likely to misdiagnose the problem and jump to psychiatric medications.

The Common Culprits of Misdiagnosis

Many disorders hover between physical and mental, thus making a correct diagnosis difficult. Several of these disorders present themselves solely as psychiatric in nature; upon diagnosis and treatment of the physical disorder, the symptoms of depression and mood disturbances usually clear up without any specific treatment for the depression. Other physical disorders present themselves at least partially as psychiatric in nature. When these conditions are successfully treated, the psychiatric symptoms clear at least partially.

The following are several of the most common physical ailments that present themselves as completely or partially psychiatric in nature and either exacerbate or cause depression.

Hyperthyroidism and Hypothyroidism

Hyperthyroidism (an overactive thyroid gland) can cause symptoms that mimic those of several mental disorders, including panic disorder, mania, neurosis and depression. Hypothyroidism (an underactive thyroid gland) can also cause symptoms that resemble those of psychiatric disturbances—in fact, one form of hypothyroidism causes symptoms that meet the DSM-IV criteria for major depression, and some studies conclude that patients with symptoms of depression should have their thyroid-stimulating hormone levels tested.

Vitamin Deficiencies

Numerous studies point to vitamin and mineral deficiencies—particularly B-vitamin deficiencies and zinc deficiencies—as principal culprits in false depressive symptoms. The symptoms of these deficiencies include paranoia, irritability, apathy, schizophrenia, fatigue, depression, weight loss, appetite loss and more. Observational evidence links high levels of homocysteine (attributed to lack of B vitamins) to various depressive symptoms, but clinical trials have not substantiated these claims.

Heavy Metal Poisoning

Heavy metal poisoning occurs chiefly from high levels of exposure to or ingestion of lead, mercury, manganese, zinc, magnesium, copper, arsenic and aluminum. Elevated levels of any of these in the body can cause a form of "brain allergy," thereby producing symptoms similar to those of psychiatric and mental illness, including major depression.

Hypoglycemia

Hypoglycemia (low blood sugar) can cause symptoms nearly identical to those of depression. Inconsistent blood-sugar levels and difficulty assimilating glucose properly usually exaggerate these symptoms, lowering physical energy levels and ultimately lowering mental and emotional levels as well.

Drugs and Alcohol

The use and abuse of alcohol and illicit drugs can cause symptoms of mental disorders. Many studies show that prescription drugs are also a principal cause of depression-like symptoms. *Prevention's New Encyclopedia of Common Diseases* quotes the *Journal of the American Geriatrics Society*, stating, "Drugs, either prescribed by a physician or taken independently, are often responsible for the development of depression, the aggravation of preexisting depression, or the production of depression-like symptoms."

Drug users commonly experience mental states that mimic major depression and other psychiatric disorders. When dealing with these patients, health care providers must perform tests to determine the extent of drug use, intoxication and withdrawal to rule out or implicate psychiatric disorders as the cause of the symptoms.

The link between drug use and depression is also a concern among the elderly. Most elderly people in the United States use prescription drugs, and most of these medications cause side effects, which may include depression.

A strong link exists between alcohol abuse and depression, and studies suggest that hypericum is effective in treating alcohol-induced depression; however, one should remember that stopping the substance abuse will at least partially alleviate the symptoms of depression.

The following are many (but not all) prescription drugs that can cause symptoms similar to those of major depression.

- anti-inflammatory drugs (Naprosyn)
- birth control pills and other hormonal medicines
- hypertension medications (Apresoline)
- heart medications
- sleeping medications (Valium)

Tumors (Cancer)

Various forms of malignant tumors have been known to cause symptoms of depression, even before physical signs of the tumor appear. Such tumors often secrete dopamine, histamine, corticotropin and serotonin, chemicals that can affect the brain and other body systems.

Nutrition

The idea that what we eat can have a profound effect on our brain chemistry and other seemingly non-related body systems has gained widespread acceptance in the medical community. The connection between depression and nutritional deficiencies, food sensitivities, allergies and poor dietary habits is inspiring more investigation into the role nutrition plays in the development and prevention of depression.

Research indicates that the most common symptoms of food allergies are headaches, fatigue and depression. Allergens cause the body to react as if it is being invaded. This inevitably affects brain chemistry and may cause episodes of mood or nervous disorders.

Other disorders that may cause depressive symptoms
- hyperadrenalism and hypoadrenalism
- mononucleosis
- hepatitis (all forms)
- multiple sclerosis

What Can You Do?

In the introduction to a compilation of articles on depression, Dr. Frederic Flach (a widely noted researcher and the author of the groundbreaking book *The Secret Strength of Depression*) stresses that depression is not necessarily its own illness; rather, it is a symptom (or group of symptoms) that the body manifests when dealing with other stresses and disturbances. He states:

"Early on [in my career], I could appreciate the complexity of depression, in which psychological, environmental and biologic factors all played significant etiological roles…in this context, I reformulated my own concept of what depression is—and what it is not. Being depressed, per se, is neither a weakness nor an illness. Rather, depression is the way healthy human beings respond to certain stresses…Depression can be viewed as an illness when it is not recognized and acknowledged, when it gets out of hand and overwhelms a client, when it persists, and—most important—when the individual cannot recover from an episode on his or her own."

Naturopathic and holistic physicians have always stressed the notion that many of today's diseases are not technically diseases—they are often bodily responses to some other underlying disorder. Symptoms disappear when the underlying cause is taken care of.

To identify any underlying physical conditions, one ought to undergo a complete physical, neurological and endocrinological examination by a professional trained in both psychiatry and internal medicine. These examinations may reveal other conditions that could cause depression. From there, a complete regimen involving physical, emotional and psychiatric aid can be implemented. Simple lifestyle changes, such as diet alterations and increased physical activity, can have profound effects on the severity, length and frequency of depressive episodes. And using natural supplements such as hypericum extract instead of harsher synthetic antidepressants can aid in the eventual recovery from depression.

Conclusion

Depression can be a devastating disorder; however, mild to moderate cases can often be successfully overcome through natural treatment and lifestyle changes, allowing for a normal and productive life. Abundant research indicates that depression is largely misdiagnosed and mistreated and that a number of alternative therapies—including St. John's wort, valerian, 5-HTP and light therapy—can help people successfully and safely overcome depression. For many people, safe, natural remedies and basic lifestyle changes may be the keys to a happy, depression-free life.

Appendix: How Do I know If I'm Suffering from Postpartum Depression?

The Edinburgh Postnatal Depression Scale (EPDS) is a helpful tool for identifying postpartum depression. Simply answer the following questions, then tally your score using the key provided at the bottom.

In the past 7 days:

1. I have been able to laugh and see the funny side of things
     a. As much as I always could
     b. Rather less than I used to
     c. Definitely less than I used to
     d. Not at all

2. I have looked forward with enjoyment to things
    a. As much as I ever did
    b. Rather less than I used to
    c. Definitely less than I used to
    d. Not at all
3. I have blamed myself unnecessarily when things went wrong
    a. Yes, most of the time
    b. Yes, some of the time
    c. Not very often
    d. No, never
4. I have been anxious or worried for no good reason
    a. No, not at all
    b. Hardly ever
    c. Yes, sometimes
    d. Yes, very often
5. I have felt scared or panicky for no good reason
    a. Yes, quite a lot
    b. Yes, sometimes
    c. No, not much
    d. No, not at all
6. Things have been getting on top of me
    a. Yes, most of the time I haven't been able to cope at all
    b. Yes, sometimes I haven't been coping as well as usual
    c. No, most of the time I have coped quite well
    d. No, I have been coping as well as ever.
7. I have been so unhappy that I have had difficulty sleeping
    a. Yes, most of the time
    b. Yes, sometimes
    c. Not very often
    d. No, not at all
8. I have felt sad or miserable
    a. Yes, most of the time
    b. Yes, quite often
    c. Not very often
    d. No, not at all

9. I have been so unhappy that I have been crying
   a. Yes, most of the time
   b. Yes, quite often
   c. Only occasionally
   d. No, never
10. The thought of harming myself has occurred to me
    a. Yes, quite often
    b. Sometimes
    c. Hardly ever
    d. Never

Scoring:

Questions 1, 2 and 4: a, 0; b, 1; c, 2; d, 3.
Questions 3, 5-10: a, 3; b, 2; c, 1; d, 0.

The maximum possible score is 30. If your score is 10 or higher, you may be suffering from depression and may wish to consult a physician or a mental health professional for more help. Question number 10 is the most important—if you have thought of harming yourself or your baby, seek help immediately. If you don't know where to turn, the following Web sites may be helpful:

www.4women.gov
www.depressionafterdelivery.com

References

Barnard, K. and C. Colón-Emeric. 2010. "Extraskeletal effects of vitamin D in older adults: cardiovascular disease, mortality, mood, and cognition." *American Journal of Geriatric Pharmacotherapy* 8(1): 4–33.

Bjerkenstedt, L. et al. 2005. "Hypericum extract LI 160 and fluoxetine in mild to moderate depression: a randomized, placebo-controlled multi-center study in outpatients." *European Archives of Psychiatry & Clinical Neuroscience* 255(1): 40–7.

Borrelli, F. and A.A. Izzo. 2009. "Herb-drug interactions with St. John's wort (*Hypericum perforatum*)—an update on clinical observations." *AAPS Journal* 11(4): 710–27.

Butterweck, V. et al. 2002. "Long-term effects of St. John's wort and hypericin on monoamine levels in rat hypothalamus and hippocampus." Brain Research 930(1–2): 21–29.

Buysse, D.J. et al. 2010. "Can an improvement in sleep positively impact on health?" *Sleep Medicine Reviews* April 26 (Epub ahead of print).

Caccia, S. and M. Gobbi. 2009. "St. John's wort components and the brain: uptake, concentrations reached and the mechanisms underlying pharmacological effects." *Current Drug Metabolism* (9): 1055–65.

Cipriani, A. et al. 2005. "Fluoxetine versus other types of pharmacotherapy for depression." *Cochrane Reviews* (4).

Conn, V.S. 2010. "Depressive symptom outcomes of physical activity interventions: meta-analysis findings." *Annals of Behavioral Medicine* April 27 (Epub ahead of print).

Coppen, A. and C. Bolander-Gouaille. 2005. "Treatment of depression: time to consider folic acid and vitamin B12." *Journal of Psychopharmacology* 19(1): 59–65.

Cox, J.L and J.M. Holden. 1987. "Detection of postnatal depression: development of the 10-item Edinburgh Postnatal Depression Scale." *British Journal of Psychiatry* 150:782–86.

Desan, P. et al. 2007. "A controlled trial of the Litebook light-emitting diode (LED) light therapy device for treatment of Seasonal Affective Disorder (SAD)." *BMC Psychiatry* 7:38.

Flach, F. 1996. "Introduction." In *The Hatherleigh Guide to Managing Depression*. New York: Hatherleigh.

Flory, R. et al. 2010. "A randomized, placebo-controlled trial of bright light and high-density negative air ions for treatment of Seasonal Affective Disorder." *Psychiatry Research* 177(1–2): 101–08.

Ford, A.H. et al. 2010. "The B-Vitage Trial: a randomized trial of homocysteine lowering treatment of depression in later life." *Trials* 11:8.

Freeman, D. et al. 2010. "Persecutory ideation and insomnia: findings from the second British Natinoal Suvey of Psychiatric Morbidity." *Journal of Psychiatric Research* April 28 (Epub ahead of print).

Freeman, M.P. 2009. "Complementary and alternative medicine (CAM): considerations for the treatment of major depressive disorder." *Journal of Clinical Psychiatry* 70(Suppl 5): 4–6.

Gagné, A.M. et al. 2010. "When a season means depression [article in French]." *Médecine Sciences (Paris)* 26(1): 79–82.

Gold, M.S. 1996. "The risk of misdiagnosing physical illness as depression." In *The Hatherleigh Guide to Managing Depression*. New York: Hatherleigh.

Guimarães, J.M. et al. 2009. "Depressive symptoms and hypothyroidism in a population-based study of middle-aged Brazilian women." *Journal of Affective Disorders* 117(1–2): 120–23.

Harsora, P. and J. Kessmann. 2009. "Nonpharmacologic management of chronic insomnia." *American Family Physician*. 79(2):125–30.

Hausman, A. et al. 2008. "Women seek for help—men die! Is depression really a female disease?" *Neuropsychiatry* 22(1): 43–48.

Heitzman, J. 2009. "Sleep disturbances—cause or result of depression." *Psychiatria Polska*. 43(5): 499–511.

Ille, R. et al. 2007. "'Add-On' therapy with an individualized preparation consisting of free amino acids for patients with a major depression." *European Archives of Psychiatry and Clinical Neuroscience* 257(4): 222–29.

Jacka, F.N. et al. 2009. "Association between magnesium intake and depression and anxiety in community-dwelling adults: the Hordaland Health Study." *Australian and New Zealand Journal of Psychiatry* 43(1): 45–52.

Kaehler, S.T. et al. 1999. "Hyperforin enhances the extracellular concentrations of catecholamines, serotonin and glutamate in the rat locus coeruleus." Neuroscience Letters 262(3): 199–202.

Kalkunte, S.S. et al. 2007. "Antidepressant and antistress activity of GC-MS characterized lipophilic extracts of Ginkgobiloba leaves." *Phytotherapy Research* 21(11): 1061–65.

Kaschel, R. 2009. "Ginkgo biloba: specificity of neuropsychological improvement—a selective review in search of differential effects." *Human Psychopharmacology: Clinical and Experimental*. 24(5): 345–70.

Laakmann, G. et al. 1998. "St. John's wort in mild to moderate depression: the relevance of hyperforin for the clinical efficacy." Pharmacopsychiatry 31(Suppl 1): 54–59.

Linde, K. 2009. "St. John's wort: an overview." *Forschende Komplementärmedizin* 16(3): 146–55.

Moncrief, J. and D. Cohen. 2005. "Rethinking models of psychotropic drug action." *Psychotherapy and Psychosomatics* 74:145–53.

Moncrief, J. and D. Cohen, D. 2006. "Do antidepressants cure or create abnormal brain states?" *PLoS Medicine* 3(7): 240.

Morin, C.M. et al. 2006. "Psychological and behavioral treatment of insomnia: update of the recent evidence (1998-2004)." *Sleep* 29(11): 1398–414.

Muscatell, K.A. et al. 2010. "Stressful life events, chronic difficulties and the symptoms of clinical depression." *Journal of Nervous and Mental Disease* 197(3): 154–60

Obach, R.S. 2000. "Inhibition of human cytochrome P450 enzymes by constituents of St. John's wort, an herbal preparation used in the treatment of depression." Journal of Pharmacology and Experimental Therapeutics 294(1): 88–95.

Papakostas, G.I. 2009. "Evidence for S-adenosyl-L-methionine (SAM-e) for the treatment of major depressive disorder." *Journal of Clinical Psychiatry.* 70(Suppl 5): 18–22.

Pinter, P. et al. 2010. "Medical clearance in the psychiatric emergency setting: a call for more standardization." *International Journal of Health Care Quality Assurance* 13(2): 77–82.

Postolache, T.T. et al. 2007. "Changes in allergy symptoms and depression scores are positively correlated in patients with recurrent mood disorders exposed to seasonal peaks in aeroallergens." *Scientific World Journal* 7:1968–77.

Resler, G. et al. 2008. "Effect of folic acid combined with fluoxetine in patients with major depression on plasma homocysteine and vitamin B12, and serotonin levels in lymphocytes." *Neuroimmunomodulation* 15(3): 145–52.

Riemann, D. 2009. "Does effective management of sleep disorders reduce depressive symptoms and the risk of depression?" *Drugs* 69(Suppl 2): 43–64.

Ross, B.M. et al. 2007. "Omega-3 fatty acids as treatments for mental illness: which disorder and which fatty acid?" *Lipids in Health and Disease* 18(6): 21.

Ross, S.M. 2009. "Sleep disorders: a single dose administration of valerian/hops fluid extract (dormeasan) is found to be effective in improving sleep." *Holistic Nursing Practice* 23(4): 253–56.

Sakakibara, H. and K. Ishida. 2006. "Antidepressant effect of extracts from Ginkgo biloba leaves in behavioral models." *Biological and Pharmaceutical Bulletin* 29 (8): 1767–70.

Sarris, J. and D.J. Kavanagh. 2009. "Kava and St. John's wort: current evidence for use in mood and anxiety disorders." *Journal of Alternative and Complementary Medicine* 15(8): 827–36.

Shaw, K. et al. 2002. "Are tryptophan and 5-hydroxytryptophan effective treatments for depression? A meta-analysis." *Australian and New Zealand Journal of Psychiatry* 36(4): 488–91.

Springhouse. 2010. *Handbook of Signs and Symptoms.* Ambler, PA: Lippincott Williams & Wilkins.

Wakefield, J.C. et al. 2010. "Does the DSM-IV clinical significance criterion for major depression reduce false positives? Evidence from the National Comorbidity Survey Replication." *The American Journal of Psychiatry* 167(3): 298–304.

Wang, Y. et al. 2010. "Hypericin prolongs action potential duration in hippocampal neurons by acting on K+ channels." *British Journal of Pharmacology* 159(7): 1402–07.

Wheatley, D. 2005. "Medicinal plants for insomnia: a review of their pharmacology, efficacy and tolerability." *Journal of Psychopharmacology* 19 (4): 414–21.